F A C I A L
S H I F T

A D J U S T I N G   T O   A N
A L T E R E D   A P P E A R A N C E

D A W N   S H A W

ISBN: 978-0-692-65979-3

DISCLAIMER

Cover Design: John Matthews and Carolyn Sheltraw
Internal Design: Carolyn Sheltraw
Editing: Kate Makled & Maggie McReynolds
Author's photo courtesy of the author, taken by AJC Photography.

DEDICATION

For David, Colleen, Tom, Crystal, Vanessa,
JR, Vernon, Brian, Pauline, John, Kathleen,
Durwood, Dean, Roland, Charlene, Barbara,
Mark, James, Brady, Aneesa, Adele, Greg
and all the other wonderful, inspiring people
I've met and interacted with in the
facial difference community.

You are living proof that what
this book is about is achievable.

TABLE OF CONTENTS

INTRODUCTION: "MY LIFE IS RUINED!"

THE EFFECT YOUR DIFFERENCE HAS ON YOUR LIFE.

Looking back, your life seemed pretty perfect. Friends, a job, living on your own, a significant other. You were well liked, and didn't lack for things to do and people to hang out with.

Then all that comfort and stability changed in an instant. Your face, once symmetrical and "normal," has been forever altered. What can be done medically to stabilize you has been done, and your physical wounds are healing or have healed. You may still have some surgeries ahead of you, but they are no longer imminent or all consuming. You are at a point at which you are confronted with having to live your life.

And you're not sure what to do.

I grew up with partial facial paralysis. Admittedly, I've had nearly five decades to adjust to my different appearance. I know what you're thinking, and in a way, you're right. Since I've never known anything different, it's hard for me to relate to someone who has to adjust to such an abrupt change. Unlike you, however, I will never know what I would have looked like without my facial difference or the condition that caused it.

More significantly, here is what we *do* have in common. How others react to our appearance is the same, whether the alteration of our physical features happened in infancy or last week. The severity of our difference doesn't seem to matter much in others' perceptions. They see us as "different," and they notice.

Our insecurities and our fears are also remarkably similar.

First, my story.

* * * * *

When I was born I could barely breathe. A growth about the size of my dad's fist protruded from the cheek and neck on my left side, interfering with my airway. My dad stands well over 6 feet tall, and even in his 80's, he sports a sturdy, robust build. So we're talking a sizable fist. Imagine that on the neck of a newborn.

I was immediately whisked away so they could insert a breathing tube into my trachea below the tumor. Only after this life-saving procedure was complete could they address the nature of the growth itself. As soon as feasible, they scooped out the contents, much as you might shell out the contents of a Halloween pumpkin. A biopsy of the material removed revealed the benign but fast-growing tumor to be a rare type called a teratoma. A teratoma is typically made up of organ tissue from other parts of the body that has congregated to one location and grown in an unusual pattern. Mine consisted primarily of brain tissue. Thankfully, there was still the requisite amount of brain tissue left in the proper place, safely encased in the crown of my skull.

Since they had carefully worked around the bone structure, nerves, and blood vessels, my face remained largely intact after the tumor's initial removal, though I did have a large, floppy flap of skin hanging down where it had been stretched by the interloper.

Just over a month later, however, the tumor grew back. This time, the medical team knew they had to be more assertive. They discovered the tumor to be intertwined with bone, nerve, and muscle, which meant that during the final removal, all that had to come out, too.

By the time they were done, I was minus many of the important structural components making up the left side of my face. My jaw was free-floating, unattached on the left side. The missing and damaged nerves not only paralyzed that side of my face, but left me with significant hearing loss in my left ear. Lack of muscle meant there was nothing to hold my facial features in place, so the corner of my mouth, the left side of my nose, and the soft tissue below my eye all droop downward, in stark contrast to the fully muscled, fully functional right side.

I went through childhood enduring taunts and often being excluded. I went through puberty and entered adulthood encountering zero interest from the opposite sex. But I wasn't totally alone. I had great support and encouragement from family and educators, and though I didn't have many friends, I had formed a handful of good, solid relationships, albeit with other "outcasts."

Reconstructive and cosmetic surgeries have gradually improved my overall appearance over the years, but the symmetry could not be restored. After a failed surgery threatened my life at age 21, I came to the inevitable conclusion that medical science couldn't "fix" my face. I was always going to look different, and determined the degree of difference mattered little. I was always going to have a face that people noticed and children stared at, and I resolved myself to learning to live with it.

But self-acceptance didn't happen overnight. It was a long, gradual process full of emotional ups and downs. I'm going to help you streamline this process.

First, however, we need to address internal stresses you may be feeling. Stresses that you might not even be aware of.

You might still be in shock. Your world has just been rocked in a violent, unanticipated and unpleasant way. You might be emotionally numb, uncertain of what to feel. Maybe you're having trouble getting your head around the idea that things will never be the way they were. You may feel overwhelmed by a sense of helplessness and unsure what to do first or next.

South African native Vanessa Carter was in a terrible car accident at the age of 24, suffering life-altering injuries to her face and body. In her essay *Six Days*, she addressed seeing herself in the mirror for the first time.

"The first time I looked at my damaged face in the mirror after the accident, I'll never forget how scared I was. I knew from the conversations around me that the damage was severe. When I finally found the courage to look, my heart sank with the realization of what had happened. The hardest part was that I had no idea how to begin fixing it. That day taught me that when something is out of your control, sometimes the only choice you have is to stop burdening your mind with panic and to try work on one small solution at a time. It took intense emotional and mental work, but to survive I had to keep my thoughts intact, let the fear go and move forward with my life. I had to accept that I wouldn't know the answers immediately. It would take time. In the meantime, I had to learn to look past my distorted face and work on what I had."

You are likely experiencing some after-effects of trauma. As a result of the many surgeries I had at a young age, I felt very uncomfortable in hospitals for many years after. The smells, sights and sounds would trigger unpleasant and vivid memories. I would tense up and had to resist the urge to just *leave*. Seeing someone with an intravenous tube inserted made me shudder and my hand would hurt in empathetic pain. I never let those feelings stop me from going to hospitals and visiting people, however, because supporting that friend or family member was more important than my own discomfort. Over time the unpleasantness faded, as it will for you as well. Since your trauma is so much more recent, be aware of the level at which your experience affects you. If you believe the intensity of your symptoms could point to Post Traumatic Stress Disorder (PTSD), seek medical help.

You may be caught up in blame. Blaming whoever caused the accident. Blaming someone you believe could have prevented it. Blaming yourself for not acting differently or just for being in the wrong place at the wrong time. Blaming others leads to anger. Blaming yourself leads to guilt. Guilt feeds anxiety and depression. None of these feelings, though completely understandable, are productive for you to keep reliving. The sooner you let go of blame, either through forgiveness or by acknowledging that knowing who's at fault doesn't alter your current situation, the sooner you will be able to start moving forward with your life.

Anyone who experiences a radical, sudden and unpleasant change in their life will need time to grieve. Just like losing a person you love, you will need to process what you have lost and how that affects your life going forward. It may be the physical attractiveness of your face, or as simple as your symmetrical sense of normalcy. Grief is a crucial process which should not be easily dismissed or ignored.

I grieve that I will never know what I might have looked like had I been born without the tumor. However, I intrinsically know that my life might have been very different, including who I made friends with, how I related to others, which talents I chose to develop, the lessons I learned and how I learned

If you ever reach the point where you start to take such thoughts more seriously and find yourself getting ready to take action, don't keep it to yourself. Talk to someone. A friend, a loved one, even a crisis hotline. Despite how it may seem sometimes, there are people who love you. It *is* possible to love yourself, even if right now you are dejected by what you see in the mirror.

If any of these fears or feelings resonate, keep reading this book. I will address each of these worries, helping you to develop resilience and to realize what your life can be: full of joy, worth and love. You are not alone. Many, such as Vanessa, David, Lizzie and myself have struggled with life-altering differences and adapted. Your appearance is only a small part of who you are. Don't let that small part control you.

CHAPTER 1:
"EVERYONE TREATS ME LIKE A FREAK!"
UNDERSTANDING THE REACTIONS OF OTHERS.

When you have a facial difference, people will generally notice. We can't help it. It's ingrained in us as a species. In the same way that understanding why we have a facial difference helps others to accept us as being human, understanding *why* people react the way they do when they see our unusual faces might help lessen the hurt we feel to be noticed in such a way. Because, *really*, it's usually not intended as a personal affront.

As human beings, we are psychologically programmed to notice and be suspicious of things that are different. It's a primitive survival trait. *Is the stranger friend or foe? Is this creature I've never seen before dangerous? Do I stand my ground or do I run (fight or flight)?*

Staring occurs because it takes our brains awhile to process the influx of new information.

In his article for *Mosaic* titled "Facial Discrimination," author Neil Steinberg writes: "Freud classified certain objects as 'unheimlich,' a difficult-to-translate word akin to 'uncanny': strange, weird, unfamiliar. Waxwork dummies, dolls, mannequins can frighten us because we aren't immediately sure what we're looking at, whether it's human or not, and that causes anxiety. A surprisingly large part of the human brain is used to process faces. Identifying friend from foe at a distance was an essential survival skill on the savannah, and a damaged face is thought to somehow rattle this system. The psychologist Irvin Rock demonstrated this in his landmark 1974 paper 'The perception of disoriented figures.' Rock showed that even photos of familiar faces—famous people like Franklin D Roosevelt, for instance—will look unsettling when flipped upside down. Just as, if you tip a square enough it stops being a square and starts becoming a diamond, so rotating a face makes it seem less like a face. The mind can't make immediate sense of the inverted features, and reacts with alarm. A bigger change, such as taking away the nose, transforms the face severely enough that it teeters on no longer seeming a human face at all, but something else."

Many reactions by other people are involuntary. For example, the double-take. In her book *Survival of the Prettiest, the Science of Beauty*, Nancy Etcoff cites: "Researcher and anthropologist, Donald Giddeon, discovered that a twenty-fifth of a millimeter discrepancy in the placement of a facial feature triggers something in the brain that causes us to do a double take."

Neil Steinberg explains: "This 'startle' reaction is a cause of much distress, both for people with disfigurements and for those they encounter, who must compress the lengthy adjustment period that recovering patients themselves go through into a moment, and tend not to do it well." To paraphrase, it takes time to adjust to something unexpected. When someone sees us for the first time, in order to be "polite," they have to squelch all the normal involuntary human reactions. This is done more successfully by some than by others, as you may have experienced already.

We expect that a face should be largely symmetrical. Nancy Etcoff notes, "As a rule, humans do not like asymmetry. When we look at someone's face, we judge beauty in large part according to how symmetric they are."

This whole asymmetry thing is one reason I quit having surgeries. I came to my own conclusion that the infinitesimal amount of difference being made in the symmetry of my face by each consecutive surgery was having little effect on people continuing to notice my difference. I instinctively knew that despite all the surgical efforts to "fix" my face, people would still stare at me and that the changes that were possible would not be significant enough for people to stop noticing. The research, of which I was completely ignorant, bears this out.

Humans are by nature curious, and often as they stare they are running an inner dialogue such as *"I wonder what happened...?"* As they attempt to process what they are seeing, they may not even realize they are staring and are embarrassed when caught.

Why is it that stares upset us so much? They make us feel objectified, as if we are an unusual artifact rather than a human being. More importantly, however, they remind us that we are different. I, for one, am not looking in a mirror or at a photo of myself 100% of the time. I'm not constantly thinking about how different I look. Mostly, I am going about the business of living my life, focusing on anything from mundane errands to the next level of achievement in my work. When we are stared at, treated in a condescending way—or worse, someone makes a rude comment about our appearance—we are abruptly and painfully reminded of our physical difference. I believe that is why those of us who have looked different for a longer period have developed psychological and behavioral filters. It's not that we aren't hurt by the reactions of others. We just don't notice them as much.

It might help to consider that people who are extremely physically attractive also receive stares, and they are also objectified. Different from us, however, is that sometimes people will fall all over them, attending to their every need in a desire to *please* them. This can be just as annoying and unwanted as the negative behavior we experience. Assumptions are made about such people, too. For example, that excessive physical beauty equates to lack of intelligence, or that someone so pretty and so smart must really have their life together, which often isn't the case. Remember, it's not how you look; rather, it's how you feel about how you look that makes the difference in how you interact with the world.

Let's expand on the human tendency toward making assumptions. Assumptions come about because we want to link uncertain things to those that are known and familiar. The reality is, however, that assumptions are just best guesses, and are often wrong. Making up something that makes sense to them rather than asking us what actually happened often makes us feel invalidated. For example, people assume that because I've obviously had an injury to my face that I was in a car accident, and that's what they tell other people who ask them about me. You can see how assumptions can contribute to the spread of rumors, which can be hurtful to us when no harm was originally intended.

Unfortunately, some people associate having a different face with having a developmental disability. This may be in part because people with Down syndrome, as well as a number of other genetic and inborn conditions resulting in developmental delay, *do* have distinctive facial characteristics. Or it may just stem from a tendency to regard anyone with any sort of difference or disability as inferior, damaged, or less capable until we prove otherwise.

In his *Mosaic* article, Neil Steinberg interviewed Randy James, who has been missing most of one ear from birth due to Goldenhar syndrome, a genetic condition that distorts the fetal face to varying degrees. "'The teachers assumed I must be stupid,' says James, who was put in a class with children who had learning disabilities—until teachers realized that he was actually very bright, only shy, and missing an ear, which made it harder for him to hear. He was allowed to sit in the front of the room, where he could hear the teacher, and his grades soared."

Due to our facial differences, some of us may have disrupted speaking abilities and are more difficult to understand when we talk. We may need to enunci-ate more, or to speak more slowly and deliberately. People erroneously associate slower speech with a slower brain. Despite this, we must insist on speaking for ourselves and try not to get too frustrated when we are not understood the first, or even second, time.

Another reason people may interpret us as less intelligent might be due to our lack of ability to exe-cute clear facial expressions. Human beings rely a lot on facial expressions to get a sense of what someone is thinking or feeling. People with paralysis issues, such as Moebius syndrome, in which major nerves in the face are either absent or non-functioning, or peo-ple like myself whose facial structure and mobility is partially affected, are unable to animate all or parts of our faces to form recognizable expressions and are therefore missing a vital communication tool. People then *might* assume because they can't read our facial expressions, we must not be feeling anything or that perhaps we are incapable of relating our feelings at all.

Regardless of the reason, such assumptions, espe-cially when vocalized, can be degrading and hurtful. Back in college, I was walking home from class one afternoon when I met up with a young boy and his mother coming out of the small dentist office next door to where I lived.

"Retard!" he yelled to my face, quite suddenly and unexpectedly.

I was so taken aback I didn't even know how to respond. I looked at him in shock, then glanced at the mother, who looked completely mortified. However, no words were exchanged as she whisked him quickly to a nearby car while I turned up my sidewalk. I regret the missed opportunity to educate, though my head wasn't in that space at the time. Moreover, the mother might not have cooperated, wishing only to get herself and her son away from a scene of such embarrassment.

There is no excuse for rude comments, but unfortunately on occasion they will happen. Sometimes it's best to walk away. Sometimes it's best to educate, especially with children. Realize, however, that depending on the parents and the situation, education is not always possible. It's easy to allow such rude behavior to affect us, and we may feel discouraged from going out in public for fear of being hurt again. But go out we must. We must endure the sting because it, too, will pass. We mustn't allow the ignorance and rudeness of others to control our behavior and stop us from living our lives.

Bullying is a whole different issue. Bullying is about power and control, not ignorance. A bully deliberately tries to make someone else feel bad in order to make themselves feel more powerful. People think of bullying as a school problem, but adults bully, too. Rude comments certainly fall under the category of bullying behavior, but so do other behaviors such as unwanted physical contact, exclusion, confinement, theft of personal property, and manipulation. In adult relationships in which one person bullies, the term "abusive" is more commonly used instead. This applies to both physical and emotional abuse. I'll dig deeper into relationship issues in later chapters.

Another common reaction from others is simple avoidance. In a few cases, this may stem from the fear that someone with a facial difference may have a contagious condition. This may seem ignorant and irrational, but encountering such an individual, who might also be germophobic, is actually quite rare. Most likely, avoidance happens because people are uncertain of how to react or respond to you. This may go hand in hand with more common assumptions or questions—assuming that because your face is different you may have a developmental disability as well, or depending on how your face is affected, being unsure of how well you are able to communicate. Talking to someone with a difference may just plain make some people uncomfortable because they do not know what to expect.

My husband Ian and I volunteer to sell merchandise for the bands we like, most commonly Carbon

Leaf and Gaelic Storm. On a couple of occasions, I've noticed someone standing near the merchandise table, waiting for Ian to help them, even though he's busy helping someone else and I am not. In those cases, I politely offer assistance and have never been turned down. I cannot say for sure that they are avoiding me. We have to be just as careful about not making assumptions about what other people are thinking and feeling. If they are reluctant to interact with me, however, I put them at ease by offering friendly engagement.

People often say things in an effort to be helpful. However, we sometimes find this helpful advice to be quite annoying instead. For me, it's when people tell me about this great plastic surgeon they know who "could really help me." First, it's the assumption that I want or need help. I gave up surgery a long time ago. Not only do I feel that the amount of difference that could be made is insignificant, but after nearly 50 years of life, my face is part of my identity. While it does not define me, it is definitely part of who I am. Changing it now, even if it were possible, would be like starting over. I've accepted my appearance, and have even learned to use it to my advantage.

Someone might start telling you about someone else they know who has some sort of facial difference or disability. They might draw comparisons, or ask if what happened to them is also what happened to you. It's easy to be put off by this, but mostly they are just trying to make conversation. They may feel they cannot ignore the obvious, yet be completely clumsy about the approach.

A person may say something to me like "You're such a beautiful person!" Or, "Beauty is only skin deep," or even, "Inner beauty is what counts." This is annoying for two reasons. First, they are basically saying my appearance isn't beautiful, and secondly, if it's someone who doesn't know me, how do they know I'm beautiful on the inside? I could be a mean, angry, resentful bitch for all they know. However, I smile and either agree with them or thank them, depending on which phrase they used.

People may treat you in a condescending way, which goes along with treating you as if you're inferior. There are many stories from people with a variety of disabilities who report that rather than addressing them directly, a person might speak to their companion, as if the person with the disability is not capable of speaking for themselves. The best response is to ignore such behavior in others. Respond politely as if the person were addressing you directly as an equal, even if you are tempted to feel you have something to prove. Recognize that not everyone has had equal experiences toward developing their own sensitivity, maturity, tact, or awareness. It isn't about you at all.

Some people will pity you. The only time this is truly damaging is if you buy into it and start feeling sorry for yourself, believing you are less capable and more pathetic. This is where you do have something to prove. You have to prove to yourself and the rest of the world that you are perfectly capable of making the most of your life by being happy and productive.

The biggest question is what sort of behavior we view as crossing the line into being *rude*, and that perception will vary to some degree by individual. However, there are some behaviors I think we can all agree on. Glaring, mocking and making deliberately hurtful or insulting comments, for example. But even then, we have to make some allowances for children.

"What happened to your face?" or "Why is your lip like that?" or "Why do you hold your mouth that way?" The last one seems to imply that this is a choice; that I'm changing the shape of my mouth on purpose.

I've lost count of the number of times I've been asked these questions. It used to upset me, and my response would be angry and defensive. When kids would stare at me, I'd glare back at them. That only stopped the stares some of the time; some would just keep staring. If they asked about my face, I'd snap back an abrupt response, such as. "*It's none of your business!"* Now, however, I use these situations as educational opportunities, because I understand that children are simply curious and usually have no idea they are being rude. I also understand that once the mystery is solved and they understand that I am just a person who looks different for a reason, they lose interest and move on. Knowledge and understanding do the most to dispel fear and ignorance.

When asked directly, I'll encourage a child to ask more politely. "I'm happy to tell you, but you have to ask me nicely." I'll coach them a little. "Try this," I suggest. "May I please ask you a question?"

"May I please ask you a question?" he repeats.

"Would you mind telling me what happened to your face?" I coach. He asks me.

"I'd be happy to tell you," I respond. "I had a tumor when I was born. Do you know what a tumor is?"

And we go from there.

In another scenario, a girl ten feet away tugs on her mother's sleeve, points at me and asks her mother, "What happened to her face?" *I got news, kid. First, I can hear you. Second, mom doesn't know.* In these cases, I usually engage neutrally.

"If you are curious about my face, I'm happy to tell you, but you'll have to ask me." Sometimes this works and I start a dialogue. Sometimes, even with the mother's encouragement, the child is too shy.

True to my word, I don't tell them unless they ask. But I remain courteous.

Sometimes a child will be looking at me, then start trying to move their mouth in such a way that it mimics the shape of mine. This is more hurtful to me than spoken words, because my mind initially perceives it as mockery. As difficult as it is, I need to step back from the temptation to be offended and realize that their action is often an investigative attempt to understand what my face is doing. Their action may, in fact, be somewhat involuntary, meaning they might not even realize they are doing it. Treating it like staring is the best solution—gently pointing out that I find the behavior hurtful and making the same offer to explain my appearance.

It may seem backwards, but sometimes people around us need reassurance *from us*. A question that comes up periodically, from adults and children alike, is along the lines of, "Does it hurt?" Or, "Are you in pain?" Fortunately, aside from periods of time during which I've been recovering from surgery, my answer is "no." Your answer might be different, but I encourage you to answer honestly but in a reassuring way. For example, "Only a little, sometimes," or, "Yes, but I'm learning to manage it." If you prefer not to say or feel it's none of their business, you can respond with something like, "I appreciate your concern, but I'd rather not talk about it." This sort of response allows you to remain polite while preserving your boundary.

Because of the lack of muscles allowing my left eye to close completely or blink properly, it sometimes tears up and drips. I periodically get asked if I am crying. I believe that such questions are generally asked from genuine empathy and concern, and deserve respectful and reassuring answers.

The bottom line is that we need to allow people to be human. We may not appreciate being stared at, and we may feel hurt or annoyed because it reminds us that we are different. For our own sake and for the sake of those around us, it is imperative that we acknowledge that this is normal human behavior. Sometimes people don't even realize they're behaving in a way that is potentially hurtful until we bring it to their attention with a smile, a nod, a verbal "hello," a wave or some combination of these. It's hard sometimes, but a positive acknowledgement is the most productive way to address this sort of reaction from others. Frequently, they become embarrassed that their behavior was noticeable, which might inspire more appropriate behavior in the future.

In her article titled *An Inside Look at Being Outside of Ordinary*, Charlene Pell, founder of Facing Forward, Inc., sums it up well. "Becoming upset or angry from strangers' stares can drain you of energy. Instead, you can become the agent for change, first for yourself, and in the process, for society."

I notice when other people have a difference, and I'm sure you do, too. Evaluate your own reactions when you see someone else who is different, and that may help you understand how others react to you. You may not like what you feel, and it may hurt to consider that some of the things you are thinking and feeling may echo what others are thinking and feeling when they see you. But once you process those feelings, they will give you insight and hopefully empathy so that you can be less resentful.

Interacting with people is a great way to take their attention away from your appearance. Charlene Pell, in developing her workshop *What to Do When People Stare*, came up with her "10 Steps to Taking Control" during social interactions with people you don't really know. Here are five of them:

- Smile whenever possible. A smile is a universal passport. There is almost an innate response to return a smile.
- Make eye contact whenever possible. It expresses interest and acknowledges the other person.
- Initiate a conversation first to control the direction of the interaction. "Is that your son on first base?"

- Direct the focus of the conversation to your environment. "Is this the first time you have attended this conference?"
- Discuss your similarities and what you have in common, not your differences. "Does your daughter also attend this school?"

Expectations play a huge role in how people interact with you. If you walk into a room expecting everyone to stare at you, that may well be the only thing you notice—the one or two people who do stare. Or you will dedicate all your attention to looking for the people who might be staring or averting their glances in order to justify your fear. However, if you walk into a room like I do—with the expectation of being treated like anyone else who is going about their business— amazingly, that is usually how people will treat you. Some people refer to it as *attitude,* but I seldom have to endure rude comments or stares, because I simply expect to be treated in a professional, respectful way. And on those rare occasions where I am treated disrespectfully, my resilience allows me to process the experience and move on. It does no good to dwell on the negative.

My goal is to help you develop that resilience so you can interact with the world in a similar manner— with poise and confidence. We can use my experience as a shortcut in the hope that it won't take you nearly as long to get where I am now!

CHAPTER 2:
"I FEEL DISFIGURED!"
REPAIRING YOUR SHAKEN SELF-IMAGE.

You may feel that your very value as a human being has been diminished by your change in appearance. Others may reinforce this by making inquiries such as, "What are you going to do now?" As if your plans must now change.

There may also be a range of normal human emotions standing in your path to recovery.

You may carry guilt, believing that what happened was somehow your fault. Maybe you survived and someone else didn't. If so, it is important to ask yourself if this was something you truly had control over. Guilt is a choice. Unless it was a deliberate act on your part for which you knew the result would harm someone else, you can choose not to feel guilty.

If you "feel disfigured," you are most likely ashamed of your new appearance. Whereas guilt is the feeling or belief that you've done something bad, shame is the belief that you *are* bad—that somehow you are less of a person.

According to author Brené Brown in her book *Daring Greatly*, "Shame is the intensely painful feeling or experience of believing that we are flawed and therefore unworthy of love and belonging."

You're not. In her writings, Brené emphasizes that we are all inherently worthy. It is a state that is neither earned nor diminished. We deserve the opportunity to make the most of our lives. We all have challenges. Some are visible, some are psychological, some are physiological. But we all make choices about how to use the skills and talents we *do* have in order to live a rich, fulfilling life.

You might also be trapped in a "victim" mentality. You may have had no control over the event that changed your appearance. It may have been forced on you, or maybe it was an accident in the truest sense of the word; a blameless, no-fault incident. People around you may refer to you as a victim, and you may find yourself using that label on yourself. You may feel entitled to justice, or a financial pay-off, and that might be totally justified because you may first need to process some events that were out of your control from the standpoint of being the actual victim. However, beware of the victim *mindset*, because that can definitely slow the psychological healing process.

Having a victim mindset means you don't have to accept personal responsibility for your situation. Exhibiting a certain degree of helplessness may seem beneficial because others are more likely to do things for you. However, if you are always caught up in thinking "poor me," you will be less likely to take risks and change your circumstances. It will be too easy to fall into patterns of behavior that keep you in a rut rather than allowing you to move forward with your life.

For about a year, I lived with a drug addict. Lonely and desperate, I was romantically attracted to him, though he made no pretense of being attracted to me. Naively thinking I could be a positive influence on his life in terms of helping him get clean, and believing that once he got to know me he'd be able to see past my face, I allowed him to move into the house I was renting. I wanted love, attention, and someone to take care of. All he wanted was an enabler, and he found a great one in me. He was emotionally abusive, saying hurtful things to me and mocking the way I spoke. He stole from me to pay his drug dealer, but still I let him stay. *Why?* Because taking care of him became more important than taking care of myself. Because it was difficult to admit to myself that I had failed to change him, and he was an expert at stringing me along. Additionally, the pain of being with him didn't seem as bad as the imagined pain of being alone.

But the whole time I was with him, I recognized that I was making choices. They weren't *good* choices, but they were mine. I took responsibility for my part in this, and never considered myself to be a victim.

Even after I asked him to move out, I still had an irrational attachment to him. It was only after he got physically violent—smashing my face with the palm of his hand while I was driving a car—that I was finally able to sever the emotional tether. About three months later, I started spending time with Ian, the man I would eventually marry. I doubt Ian would have been attracted to me if I'd been wallowing in self-pity and victimhood.

Changing the victim mindset involves recognizing that you have choices. It requires you to take responsibility for your life going forward, even if what happened to you wasn't your fault.

Keep in mind the Golden Rule: *Do unto others as you would have them do unto you.* Hopefully, that includes treating others with kindness and respect. Not only is how you treat others important, but how you treat *yourself* is significant as well. The words you choose to describe yourself can make a huge difference in self-perception, and in turn, the way others perceive you.

For example, I maintain a strong objection to the use of the term "disfigured" because it has such negative connotations. People with facial differences tend to have issues with self-image, so it stands to reason that using a negative term to describe us, and expecting us to use that term to describe ourselves, is detrimental to our positive self-image.

One definition of *disfigurement* is "an appearance that has been spoiled or misshapen."

That is certainly not how I think of myself. The word *deformed* is even worse. It is defined as "to spoil the appearance of something and make it ugly," and "change for the worse in something's appearance." If I were to describe myself to others, I wouldn't say "My face is misshapen." Or deformed. Or disfigured. Or spoiled. Or flawed. Because I honestly don't feel that way about my face.

I only use these or similar terms if I am directly quoting a source; for dramatic impact; or if I am trying to make a particular point. In fact, I find it painful to read materials in which people liberally use these words to describe themselves.

So what words might be friendlier to our self-esteem?

I prefer the term "facial difference." Definitions of *difference* include "the element or factor that separates or distinguishes," or "a characteristic that distinguishes one from another or from the average." I kind of like that. I've always preferred not to be average, and instead of being described as *flawed*, I am *distinctive.*

Changing Faces, an organization in the UK that offers support services and advocates legally for people with facial differences, explains their use of the term "disfigurement" as follows: "We use 'disfigurement' as a collective word for all the conditions, scars or marks that make a person's face or body look unusual. Many people, understandably, prefer to specify their condition, for example, 'I have a birthmark'. But disfigurement is an important collective term and is used in the UK's Equality Act 2010, protecting people from discrimination." They also expressed to me that "disfigured" doesn't have as much of a negative cultural connotation in Europe. Admittedly, it does make the language very clear about whom they help and advocate for in the world and to whom the legislation applies.

When Changing Faces CEO James Partridge appeared as a guest on my *Friending the Mirror* webinar series, I asked him if he considered himself to be disfigured. He said that no, he did not. I don't consider myself to be disfigured either. [Find a link to the interview with James and view the complete list of webinar episodes at www.facinguptoit.com/

webinar.] During a discussion regarding terminology on social media, someone posted a comment saying "I feel disfigured." This did not sound like a person who is at peace with their appearance. My heart went out to them, and it made me wonder: *Is "disfigured" a state of mind?*

Then again, there are people with facial differences who are very well adapted to their appearance and continue to use the term to describe themselves. Who am I to tell them what words to use? Despite respecting everyone's right to choose their own words, I still object to the terms "disfigured" and "disfigurement." I actually trip over these words when I try to apply them to describing a human being.

What it comes down to is this: *How does the word make you feel when you read it or hear it used to describe your situation?* If it makes you feel insecure, like less of a person, or is hurtful, I recommend avoiding it and encouraging those around you to quit using it as well.

When "different" is not descriptive enough, as Changing Faces suggested, I recommend resorting to the medical condition. For example, in my case, "My face is half paralyzed." Someone with Moebius syndrome might say, "the nerves in my face are missing (or don't work)." Others could say, "My face was badly burned." Or scarred. Or injured in an accident. Whatever the facts or diagnosis may be.

If you *must* use a word like *disfigured*, I recommend only using it to describe a part of you, as in "my face is disfigured," or "I have a disfigurement," rather than "I am disfigured."

As you grieve the loss of your "normal" face, you will undoubtedly have moments when you feel relatively worse about your new appearance. No one can tell you how to grieve, just as you cannot tell yourself, or others, for that matter, how to feel. Allow yourself to experience the full ranges of those feelings. You don't need to put on a brave front for friends and family. In fact, expressing your true feelings to others can be helpful for all involved.

Don't be discouraged if you seem to be coping all right and then *BOOM!* you find yourself in the emotional dumps again. Even though I consider myself well-adjusted, I still have days when I feel less confident and secure about my appearance. There are still times I want to hide away or tear my whole face off and start over.

* * *

As I walked out of the veterinary office, a young blond boy stared at me. I said "hi" to him in an effort to diffuse his curiosity, and to show that I am a real, responsive person. He shyly said "hi" back to me. *Good.*

His mother and an older boy who was taller but otherwise a spitting image were still at their car. I said "hello" cordially as I passed. The mother carried a small terrier wrapped in a towel. She returned the greeting politely but without enthusiasm.

However, as I walked away, I heard the youngest boy behind me.

"Did you see her?"

I bristled and slowed my step, but waited. I wanted to be sure…

"Did you see her?" he repeated. I imagined that he was talking to his brother. Then a third time. Then, "Did you see her face?"

That's it. I turned.

"Yes, he probably did see me," I replied earnestly. "If you have a question for me, you are welcome to ask me." My tone was not as welcoming as I'd have preferred.

"OK," came the quick reply from the mother, as if cowed or perhaps embarrassed by the confrontation. I grimaced. I wasn't talking to her. She was not the one who should have been responding.

"I am not deaf," I added curtly, and returned hastily to my truck.

As I drove away, rattled by the exchange, I wondered idly if putting a gun to my head and pulling the trigger wouldn't be such a bad idea after all. So much for coping. You would think I'd be used to it, but sometimes stoicism goes out the window.

Thinking about suicide does not make you suicidal. Would I ever actually attempt it myself? I doubt it. The expanse between thought and action can be quite broad. As close as I've come to death and fought to survive, suicide would be the ultimate hypocrisy.

Was my response the best way to handle the situation? Likely not, but I'm not sure that ignoring it and walking away would have been better. If such an incident were to happen today, I would most likely be less defensive and more apt to try turning it into a teachable moment. As it was, I hope the mother at least talked to her son about the situation, but in this case I somehow doubt it. So the child learned nothing positive from either of us.

At the very least, if you're going to talk about me, wait until I am out of earshot.

It should not be too much to ask to be looked upon and treated like a normal human being. Nor should it be too much to expect parents to raise their children to respect others, to be sensitive to the feelings of others, and not meekly turn away when confronted with the noticeable gaps in the experiences they have given their children to date. But changing society is a long process. In the meantime, we have to make the best of it.

Sometimes the stresses of a traumatic change in your life will have unexpected physical manifestations. You may develop anxiety-related habits you never had before, like biting your nails, cheek or lip; sleep deprivation; or picking at hair or skin. You may struggle at first with managing these new attributes or undesired results.

When I was in high school, I began plucking my eyebrows with my fingernails. At first it seemed harmless enough; I had thick eyebrows, so I had plenty to spare. Eventually, however, I developed bald spots which I'd fill in with eyebrow pencil. As time passed, those bald spots expanded to half or more of my eyebrows needing to be drawn in, leaving only tufts on either side of my nose. It was a compulsion that would last for 30 years. I tried a number of things to stop it, including covering my eyebrows with hats or band-aids, or wearing gloves, but nothing worked. I was ashamed of my lack of willpower; embarrassed by my inability to control this self-destructive activity.

Yet the absence of my eyebrows didn't stop me from going out in public. I figured that my face was enough of a detraction, who would notice that half my eyebrows were painted on? I did have some degree of vanity, however. I always carried an eyebrow pencil with me in case one got rubbed off.

I didn't talk about the eyebrow pulling very much, nor did I seek help in trying to quit. I thought I was the only one doing it. It wasn't until I'd written my memoir that my editor pointed out to me that what I thought was a bad habit unique to me had a name: *trichotillomania*, or compulsive hair pulling. It was an obsessive-compulsive disorder, which didn't surprise me at all.

Learning it had a name was a revelation. *It meant that I wasn't alone*, and that was comforting. Thinking about it, how silly to think that I'd be the only one with this sort of habit, but it's an easy mindset to get into. Unfortunately, there weren't many solutions offered either. Yet knowledge is power.

By now, I have been able to pretty much stop and my eyebrows have almost completely grown back, but this has only been a recent development. While I partially credit a simple substitution of habits, such as using an object as a diversion to occupy my needy fingers, I believe my ability to control the impulsion came primarily from inside. A few years ago, as I finished writing my memoir *Facing Up to It* and strove toward becoming a professional motivational speaker, I realized that I would be a lot more effective if I made some internal changes.

I've struggled with negativity for most of my life. I held onto anger about my situation because of the demeaning or dismissive way others sometimes treated me. My humor tended to be dark, self-deprecating and often took jabs at others. I said what I thought, sometimes without consideration of others' feelings. My outlook was often pessimistic, and I projected a brooding intensity.

However, if I was going to convince others that they could live happier lives, I needed to walk the talk. I concentrated on pushing away negative feelings and reactions and invoked a more optimistic view. I used affirmations and a vision board to help me focus on what I wanted to attract to my life. It takes time, practice and effort. While I have not magically transformed into someone who is positive and sunny all the time—I firmly believe that such an absolute would be unhealthy, not to mention impossible—I have certainly improved the positivity of my life and become overall a happier person.

If I can overcome much of the anger and negativity I'd held onto for so long, I have every confidence that you can, too. As for my self-destructive hair pulling habit; like alcoholism, there is no "cure." I am constantly fighting the temptation, and I slide now and then, sacrificing a few hairs to mindless obsession. But what stops me from regressing completely is reminding myself how hard it was to grow those eyebrows back.

I never want to go back to the way I was: angry, insecure, and lacking eyebrows.

Even though you are probably physically stable at this time, and the physical scars have mostly healed, you're going to be faced with decisions about having more surgery. This may come from medical professionals convinced they can do more to help you, from family members who expect to see your original face fully restored, or from your own desire to regain as much of your original appearance as possible. People will point to the latest medical breakthroughs such as face transplants and 3D bioprinting, both of which have been getting a lot of press lately. They will be curious about whether these might provide a viable option for you. Advances in the materials used and the much more realistic appearance of prosthetics make them a more attractive option when applicable, such as replacing part of an ear.

Regardless of whether the suggestions come from a medical professional or a well-meaning friend, research your surgical options. Are you even a viable candidate? It's up to you to educate yourself about the physical limitations of just what can be "fixed" and what can't. Then you must weigh the physical and financial costs against the range of possible results.

By cost, I am not just talking money. I'm referring to the brutality that surgery puts your body through, and the psychological toll associated with incurring pain and suffering. Make sure you are clear on the limitations and possible side effects of each procedure, as well as the odds of success and the potential negative results associated with complications or failure. What does success look like to *you*, as opposed to what your surgeon considers to be a successful outcome? Make sure your expectations are realistic. As I was growing up, I kept expecting to see huge improvements in my face after each surgery, once the swelling went down. I believed that the doctors could eventually completely "fix" me and make me look "normal" again. While improvements were made, they certainly did not approach restoring the symmetry my face needed to achieve "normalcy."

I am sure that the doctors never told me they could achieve the perfection I was looking for, and I'm not sure why I held onto this disillusionment for so long.

In 1987, I elected for a surgical procedure that would transfer fatty tissue (an omental flap) from my abdomen to my left cheek. This was an attempt to add contour to the flattened, bony left side of my face, which lacked muscle development and movement. After the procedure, I woke up in intensive care with a tube down my throat to keep my airway from swelling shut. The agony I suffered was intense, especially when the nurse would inject water into the breathing tube in order to clean it, which made me feel like I was drowning. As if that wasn't enough, the next day the newly inserted omental flap had to be removed due to severe infection. To add insult to injury, the incision down my belly, where the flap had come from originally, caused me discomfort for about a year.

After I had physically recovered, I did confer with the surgeon about further options. Rather than proceeding, however, I made the decision that enough was enough. The small, incremental improvements to my appearance from these procedures were proving not to be worth the risk, let alone the physical and emotional pain and suffering I'd been enduring. As pointed out earlier, it doesn't take much asymmetry for people to notice that your face isn't "right." I resolved that I would just have to learn to accept my appearance as it is, and I have not had any surgery related to my facial difference since.

The decision to stop having cosmetic surgery didn't exactly mean that I instantly accepted my appearance. I didn't wake up the next morning proclaiming my love for myself and giving the finger to anyone who couldn't accept me for who I was. It's been a long, hard road, and even though I'm much closer, I'm still not 100% of the way there.

I have lost count of the number of times I've been asked if I plan to have more surgery. I've even had people refer me to a plastic surgeon they know who "is wonderful and might be able to help me." This continues to happen, even to this day.

Any surgeries I do from here on out will be to improve a quality of life issue rather than an appearance issue. For example, if there was something they could do so that my left eye would blink properly and not water so much. Or if something that is working fine now starts to cause pain or give me trouble in the future. Or if they could restore normal hearing in my left ear. Then I might consider more surgery to be worthwhile. Otherwise, I'm fine the way I am.

When it comes to repairing self image, it is a multilayered process that takes *time*. Allow yourself to go through the grieving process. Acknowledge your feelings, and don't bottle them up.

Learn how to accept compliments. Having someone tell you that you are a beautiful person may sound hollow, but instead of dismissing it, say "thank you."

Focus on the things that make you feel good about your life. There must be activities you used to enjoy doing that you can still do. In fact, your altered appearance need not change the plans you had for your life. Regardless of what anyone else believes your capabilities to be, do not lower your own expectations of what you are able to accomplish. Your efforts may be delayed, or may need to be redirected, but certainly not abandoned.

What are you grateful for? Hopefully one thing you are grateful for is that you're still alive, though at times you may have mixed feelings about that. Another might be the friends and family that have supported you.

Treat yourself with respect, whether it's by allowing yourself to grieve, letting go of guilt, or choosing positive words to describe yourself.

Be careful about allowing family pressures and expectations to influence your choices about surgery. Remember, it's your pain and suffering, not theirs.

When it comes to elective surgery, Changing Faces sums up my thoughts quite well. On their web site, they cite their position on face transplants. Under the sub-heading Media Representation and Coverage, they state the following:

> "Changing Faces continues to be concerned about the way in which some parts of the British and international media occasionally portray face transplants as some kind of miracle 'fix' for all people with disfigurements. We will continue to challenge over-simplistic media coverage which:
> (a) suggests wrongly that people can't lead

happy lives unless their disfigurement is removed

(b) reinforces the stereotypical view that a disfigurement is undesirable and disastrous

(c) suggests that a public attitudes shift on disfigurement is either impossible or unnecessary."

I believe in points a, b and c above. I believe you can live a happy fulfilling life despite your facial difference. I believe that the more of us who go out there and prove this, the more there will be a societal shift toward acceptance.

I'm not saying it's easy. There will be setbacks. But the sooner you believe that these things are possible, the sooner you will stop *feeling* "disfigured."

CHAPTER 3:
"MY FRIENDS AND FAMILY DON'T WANT TO BE SEEN WITH ME."
AVOIDING SOCIAL ISOLATION.

You've seen the way your friends and family look at you. You've seen their expressions, perhaps when they thought you weren't looking. You can tell it's difficult for them to gaze upon your injured face. You witness them searching your features, trying to make sense of the situation, trying to recognize your former countenance, and thinking unknown thoughts. Some of them don't seem to be able to look you in the eye.

You are embarrassed about how you look. You envy those whose faces are still intact and symmetrical. You wish it had been anyone else but you, but you are also ashamed for thinking that way because you wouldn't wish what you've been through on anyone else, either.

You are feeling very alone. Though some of your friends and family have been supportive, visiting you in the hospital and keeping in touch, there is a distance between you. They cannot possibly understand what you are going through. The intense physical pain. The poking, prodding and invasive procedures of the hospital staff. The agony of looking in the mirror for the first time. No one could have prepared you for that.

You are frustrated at your own helplessness. You are angry at the people who don't come around anymore, hurt that they would abandon you in your hour of need. You're wondering when everyone else will abandon you, too, and the thought terrifies you. Yet you are so afraid of rejection that without realizing it, you may be pushing people away who are willing and able to support and accept you. It may be profoundly difficult to relate to the people who knew you "before." At the same time, it isn't easy to relate to the people who are coming into your life because of these new challenges. You are no longer sure where you belong and how you fit in.

Chances are, there are people in your life who love you unconditionally. Maybe it's your spouse, parents, an aunt, a sibling, or a close friend. Try not to take these people for granted. While they may not realize it, even they are there for you by choice.

There will be people in your life who either cannot handle or do not want to handle your change, and they will cease coming around or contacting you. Depending on the relationship you think you had, this could be very painful and certainly justify in your mind the feeling that "no one" wants to be around you anymore.

Here's the thing. Anyone who cares about you for the right reasons—because they enjoy your company—will still be there. *You are still YOU.*

What can you do to ward off or dispel that sense of abandonment? What can you do to avoid social isolation?

For one, reassure the people in your life that regardless of the physical change that has taken place, the real you is still inside. Here's an analogy you may find helpful:

James Partridge, a burn survivor and the founder and CEO of Changing Faces, wrote a book called *Changing Faces; the Challenge of Facial Disfigurement*, after which his non-profit organization is named. He compared having a permanently altered face to the experience of developing relationships with the hospital staff of the burn unit. The staff had to wear sterile masks to be around him, so all he could see were their eyes. During months of recovery, he built trust and relationships with people whose whole faces he'd never seen.

"You have accepted and related to all these masked people over the weeks and months of hospitalization. You have learned to read their mood and reactions by the look in their eyes or the lines on their forehead. The faces covered up by the masks are irrelevant at the time. They could even have been disfigured. What matters is their laughter, the light in their eyes, their care, advice and encouragement. As a disfigured person, you have to wear the mask of disfigurement like a hospital mask: make sure that your mask does not obscure or dim your real self. If anything, you have to make your real self that much more conspicuous... In other words, you have to come out of your introspection and adopt a new, more outgoing posture."

Think of yourself as wearing a permanent mask. It doesn't change who you are, unless you allow it to. This analogy also emphasizes the importance of presenting a positive attitude, even if sometimes it is hard to feel. *You* need to set the example for the people around you.

For people who knew you as you looked before, the change will be difficult. While trying to be supportive, they will be going through a range of their own emotions. Your attitude will drive how they approach you, because above all they will want to be responsive to your needs and feelings.

They might be feeling guilty, either because it could have been them and not you, or because they are glad it was you and not them, and they might be ashamed of feeling that way. Just as you need time to emotionally adjust to your altered appearance, they need time as well. Give them that time and be grateful that they are willing to go through this adjustment with you.

They might be uncertain as to the right thing to say, so they don't say anything. For that reason, they might avoid talking to you or coming to see you. That "outgoing posture" that James refers to means that you might be the one needing to initiate social situations. Instead of waiting to be invited, ask a friend or relative if they'd like to get coffee or do lunch. Or just call them on the phone to talk. Let them know that you still enjoy their company and want them in your life. Talk about the normal stuff you always used to talk about. Break the ice, and assure them through action that they don't need to be the one to carry the relationship through the unknown.

A few people may seem overly happy and optimistic, either because they genuinely believe that once the doctors are through, your face will be back to normal; or because they feel it is their responsibility to lighten the mood or illuminate possibility. It may take even longer for family and friends to realize the practical limits of your facial recovery than it did for you. While at some point it is important to help them understand the truth about the limitations of modern medicine, enjoy the levity and thank them for making your day a little brighter.

There are also those who will pity you, but as James wrote in his book *Changing Faces*, "...sympathy may allow or even encourage an inward-looking and self-pitying attitude on your part that can have an insidious and undermining effect on your recovery." Be careful how much influence you allow from people who have a limiting or negative outlook, whether about your face or about life in general.

James also recommends sharing your problems and concerns with family and those close to you, and seeking their advice. This helps them feel included and draws them close. There is nothing like a crisis to bring people together.

However, he cautions, "...this closeness should not become excessively protective. Sooner or later—and preferably sooner—the disfigured person has to venture out into the world freed from, but buoyed up by, family commitment. Unfortunately, there are examples of disfigured people, especially children, who have become so sheltered from the public gaze by apparently well-intentioned parents or family that they never make the transition to wearing their new face with confidence. This is something that can be achieved only by wearing it in public."

Inviting a friend or relative to go with you to a public setting such as a restaurant, movie or concert can have an unexpected side benefit. Once you start going out into the world, being with someone who has a "normal" face can act as a shield and bring you more acceptance in a social or crowd situation. Says James about outings he would take with a particular friend: "...I hid behind his normalcy and enjoyed the social acceptance that being with him brought to me. Other friends have played similar roles in many circumstances, although I did not ask them to do so, and it is unlikely they appreciated the help they were giving me."

However, there have been occasions when I've been out with a friend or relative, and they've observed people staring at me. This is where *you* get to set the example.

"That guy over there is staring at you."

"Oh, I hadn't noticed," I responded truthfully, deliberately resisting the temptation to look his direction.

"I want to go punch him!"

"What would that solve?" I queried.

On one hand, I was flattered that my companion felt so protective of me. On the other hand, when it comes to my appearance, I subscribe to the philosophy of "what I don't know won't hurt me," and am just as happy to continue my business in ignorance of curious gazes. If I had noticed this particular gentleman, I would likely have smiled and waved at him. This is one of my favorite responses; a polite way of letting him know he'd been "caught" staring.

It's always better to have a sense of humor about your situation whenever possible. It will put people at ease, and make you more fun to be around. Two cautions here, however: first, be careful that your humor is not too self-deprecating. Occasionally this is fine, but remember, no one wants to hear you constantly put yourself down, even if it is in the guise of jest. Also, keep in mind that this is humor they can't participate in. If you make a joke about your appearance, it may seem funny to you, but they might understandably be afraid to laugh with you. If someone else makes a joke about your appearance, it's going to be offensive, and rightly so. The second caution is to make sure you're not using humor to mask your true feelings. Just do a Google search to learn how many comedians have committed suicide.

When it comes to the people you care about, keep in mind that relationships can be compared to bank accounts. The "emotional bank account" metaphor is generally attributed to author Stephen Covey, though I personally learned about it from Magnús Lárusson, an Icelandic instructor who taught me much of what I know about riding and training Icelandic horses. In the horse world, a withdrawal would be realized by scaring the horse, being mean or unfair to it, or insisting it do something that it doesn't understand. A deposit would be realized by a food reward, or in any way making a training or riding session a positive experience for the horse. A horse that wants to please you and enjoys your time together is a much more pleasant horse to work with as compared to a horse that is afraid of you, or is constantly frustrated due to lack of clear communication between you. The bottom line, with either horses or people, is that it is important to keep a positive balance in the relationship.

For people, deposits into an emotional bank account may include being fun to be with, praise and gratitude, paying for lunch, listening to a friend who needs to vent, and asking for and valuing that person's opinion. However, withdrawals might include constantly being the one to vent, complaining, asking for favors, or making someone feel taken for granted. Really big withdrawals would be made in instances of verbal abuse, bullying, or taking advantage of a friend or relative without offering anything in return. You can get away with a certain amount of withdrawals—even some big ones—if the total deposits made remain larger than the withdrawals.

Sometimes, what might at first seem like a deposit may later be seen as disingenuous. For example, if one were to shower an individual with compliments for the sole purpose of "buttering up" in order to garner favors from them, eventually that person will see through it and become resentful.

In cases of extreme need, many friends and family members will rise to the occasion, even if the emotional bank account has run quite low. They will put themselves out to be there and to help, understanding that exceptional circumstances may prevent the appropriate reciprocity or prompt some out of character behavior.

While my friend Karen was dying from cancer, I did what I could to be there for her. Her husband had died several years previously, so she was a widow and nearly alone in the world. The chemo was really hard on her. I used to come visit often. Ian and I would help with minor repairs and technical needs around the house. She had a couple of horses, and we'd come periodically to help with horse chores, especially when she'd get behind.

I talked to Karen almost daily, but after awhile she became more cold toward me. I knew she was suffering, so I ignored the chill as best I could. I wanted to prove to her that I would be there for her regardless. I'd heard her lament how friends and family had abandoned her, not able to handle being around someone who was "sick," and I didn't want to be counted among those. Yet she kept pushing me away, finally telling me outright that she didn't want me around anymore.

We'd been very close, and the rejection hurt me deeply. I understood rationally that people who are dying try to make their world smaller, but I didn't think she would choose me to exclude from hers. However, rather than fighting to continue swimming upstream, I let go. I honored her wishes, as much as it pained me to do so. I'd taken a lot of abuse from her. I had allowed her to overdraw her emotional account with me because I knew she was suffering, and I thought that above anything else she needed a friend. In many respects, letting go of that relationship made my life easier, even if a part of me always felt like I'd failed her somehow.

Some people will not be as persistent as I was with Karen. Their tolerance for what they perceive as abuse may be a lot smaller. The reality is this, however, and I came to realize it through Karen. No matter how lousy you feel or what you are going through, there is no excuse for abusing the people who love you. We are not perfect all the time. Sometimes we slip and behave badly, but the occasional slip is but a small withdrawal from that person's account. But if every time we are with someone we are pushing or exceeding the boundaries of tolerance, the withdrawals might well land us in the red sooner rather than later.

Eventually, maintaining the relationship becomes too draining for the person whose account has been overdrawn. While they may give you some slack because of what you've been through, people do not want to be around someone who is negative *all* the time, or someone who is constantly exhibiting destructive behavior such as self-deprecation, victimhood, blame, bad-mouthing other people, excessive sarcasm, or lashing out at those around them. That's not to say that in order to have friends, one needs to exhibit a rosy and sunny disposition constantly and never show that they're hurting. Instead, it comes back to keeping a positive balance in that emotional bank account.

Unfortunately, rather than say something to you, friends will sometimes just melt away, because they are reluctant to confront your behavior and don't want to hurt your feelings. They don't want to be perceived as rejecting you, nor do they want to accelerate the conflict. They are afraid they would be adding emotional pain on top of the physical damage that has already been done. It is also possible that your friends don't have the flawless, mature social skills that would help you both be productive about the conflict. What they fail to realize, however, is that by backing away and *not* saying something, they leave you hurt and bewildered. Growing up, I would say things that were hurtful to my friends, only I didn't realize the degree to which they were hurtful. No one corrected me, because they figured "I'd been through so much" they didn't want to inflict more pain. They would be angry and resentful, and yet not tell me. There were a lot of social skills I failed to develop in a timely way, and some hard, painful lessons I had to learn much later in life as a result. In the meantime, I lost friendships and felt abandoned, and didn't fully understand why.

Be cognizant, not only of the status of your accounts with other people, but their respective account statuses with you. Just as you don't want to drag your friends and family down, be careful that—especially during this fragile period of emotional recovery—other people are not dragging you down.

If you are dealing with serious psychological issues alongside your facial changes, such as depression or PTSD, please don't hesitate to get help. Being down sometimes is normal, and no one expects you to be upbeat all the time, especially with the emotional and physical pain you've been enduring. But try not to take it out on the people who love you, and at the same time, try to discern whether someone else may be leading you into a negative theme unnecessarily. Own your feelings, and move through them, and don't take on other people's baggage.

I encourage you to seek out support groups so that you can interact with people who have been through what you are going through, as well as offer support to friends and family members who are seeking a better understanding of your situation. Hospitals and burn centers may have recommendations, or you can search for a Meet-Up group in your area. Facebook has several discussion groups, including the Adults with Facial Differences Networking Community, and a group I started called the Physical Differences Support, Discussion and Advocacy Group. AboutFace, an organization based in Ontario, Canada, hosts monthly support calls. They also run several camps annually where people can meet in person. There is no membership requirement, and they are very welcoming to people of any nationality. Facing Forward hosts monthly calls as well as having resources available on their web site. The Phoenix

Society for Burn Survivors hosts an annual conference and also has resources available on line. In the United Kingdom, Changing Faces provides support for people with facial differences as well as advocates for legal protection, and many of their online support materials are helpful to people anywhere in the world. You can find any of these organizations by doing an online search, or I've included their web addresses in the Resources section at the end of this book.

The most important thing to remember through this experience is that you are not alone. The friends and family who care about you will still be there, and there are many people who have been through similar experiences who are happy to offer guidance, camaraderie, and support. Embrace the people who love you unconditionally. Thank the people who spend time with you. As much as we'd like to believe we can handle things on our own, the reality is that we thrive even more with love and support from others, no matter how strong or capable we are.

CHAPTER 4:
"NO ONE WILL
LOVE ME."
NAVIGATING ROMANTIC RELATIONSHIPS.

I'm ugly now. How can anyone love me?

Unfortunately, I've heard about relationships that don't survive the physical and emotional trauma of an accident. There are people who can't handle the responsibility of being around someone who, at least for awhile, has medical needs or may require extra support both physically and emotionally. There are people who cannot handle supporting someone through adverse change, whether it is their physical appearance, their career, or their family that has suffered a loss.

Seeing a loved one go through a painful process of physical change isn't easy. Supporting my husband through his open-heart bypass surgery was highly stressful and incredibly draining, and I wasn't even the person experiencing the medical procedures. After his hospital stay, I spent several weeks in a caregiver capacity for him, as he was limited in what he was allowed to do. But I love him and I wanted to be there for him. Plus I knew without a doubt that at the drop of a hat he'd do the same for me if I ever needed it.

Understandably, you're worried about how your altered appearance will affect your ability to either stay in or find a new romantic relationship. The bottom line is this: If someone truly loves you, they will stay with you through thick and thin. If someone is truly attracted to you as a person, your face won't matter.

If your current partner leaves you because you are no longer "good-looking," then, as painful as it is, you really need to consider that person's motivations for being with you in the first place. You deserve someone who loves you for the person you are on the inside rather than how appealing your external appearance might be.

Easier said than done, you say? You will find yourself wondering, *How will I ever attract anyone else?*

You can. And you will.

· · · · · ·

There was one thing I always knew growing up. As soon as I was old enough to even think about being in a romantic relationship, I knew there was someone out there who would be able to look past my flawed face and love me for who I am. I am not sure where that belief came from. I also can't say I never doubted it, but it was instilled in me as a fundamental belief. Granted, finding that special someone wasn't easy, but in all fairness, finding the right match is hardly ever easy. When puberty struck, no one among my peers was interested in having me as a girlfriend. There were guys I had crushes on, but outside of being friends, there was no reciprocation. With these particular individuals, appearance may not have been the only factor. One of them was gay, for example. There were personality and compatibility issues to consider as well. I wasn't always a bright, sunny, upbeat person myself. I could be brooding and moody—not exactly fun to be with. Yet I was smart, honest, creative and devoted, so not completely devoid of positive attributes.

Much of the general lack of interest I chalked up simply to immaturity. Of course appearance would be a primary motivator, if not *the* primary motivator, for many young males who are just discovering their sexuality. That was one of several reasons I couldn't wait to get out of high school, because I figured once

I went to college, I would be an adult among adults. While I was correct in that I was much more broadly accepted, I drew a blank romantically there as well.

When I finally did enter into relationships, at first they were with significantly older men. However, contrary to what one might think, these men became my friends prior to a mutual decision to take the relationship to a more intimate level. Despite the age difference, I never felt that these men were taking advantage of me. Even though I fundamentally understood that because we were differently situated, it would be better all the way around if these relationships were temporary, it felt really good to have men interested in me sexually. More importantly, these relationships gave me confidence. If these men could become interested for the "right" reasons, eventually I would find a potentially more permanent partner.

These initial relationships helped me develop in another necessary way. Because of my lack of relationship experience as a teenager, I was emotionally immature. During my first sexual relationship, I was a clingy, emotional wreck. I would never have imagined that being in a relationship would take practice, but then, I also understand that you can't rationalize your way out of your underlying emotions. However, it is just as well that my first sexual relationship was never meant to last. Looking back at how I behaved, I feel sorry for him as well as grateful for the experience.

But still you are wondering, *How do I meet someone?*

Joining an online dating site is a popular way to meet potential partners in this digital age. Perhaps that scares you, and you may be thinking: *But I can't post a photo! That'd be an instant turn-off!*

Because I have been happily married for over twenty years, I have never tried online dating. However, the discussion did come up with one of my *Friending the Mirror* webinar guests: Roland, who has Moebius syndrome. Moebius syndrome involves either the inactivity or absence of the major nerves that control facial movement. People with Moebius syndrome, therefore, lack the ability to use facial expression to convey emotions. That certainly doesn't mean they don't *feel* emotion. It can be challenging for unaffected people to understand and interact with a person with facial paralysis at first, because emotional and nonverbal expression is such an integral part of how we communicate, but people afflicted in such a way are able to find other ways to express themselves.

Roland had been married for a time. As marriages sometimes do, however, his dissolved for reasons not at all related to his appearance. When seeking a new potential partner, Roland decided to try online dating. When he set up his profile, he decided to include a photograph. In his introduction, he stated very clearly that his face looked the way it did due to having Moebius syndrome, and he offered a brief explanation as to what exactly that entailed. He had a couple of responses. The first didn't pan out, primarily because she totally ignored his explanation and wrote merely to tell him he looked "sad." The second woman who responded accepted his explanation and agreed to meet with him. As of this writing, the two of them are still dating and it seems to be a good match. [Find a link to the interview with Roland and view the complete list of webinar episodes at www. facinguptoit.com/webinar.]

I am in favor of disclosure. When you are open and honest about the reasons for your appearance, it takes curiosity, and speculation, off the table. People are much more likely to accept what they understand. That's just human nature.

I also believe that it is easier for men who have a difference to find a romantic partner than it is for women. While of course women will notice a physical difference, I think it is easier for us to get past it because ultimately we are more attracted to the character of a person.

Of course, that doesn't mean finding a man able to overlook a physical difference is impossible.

However, I do believe that providing the opp[...] for people to get to know you becomes a more[...] cial factor. Considering online options, an interact[...] social media setting such as Facebook might allow a relationship to be created more organically without the pretense of being on a "dating" site.

However, there is no substitute for getting out and meeting people—in person. Whatever things you like to do, and whatever sorts of activities you enjoy, I suggest that you get out and do them, because that is where you are most likely to meet like-minded people whose interests and availability to pursue those interests most mirror your own.

Even if you believe that finding someone will be difficult due to your appearance, it is important to keep in mind that you deserve someone who loves you and who will treat you well.

Be careful not to allow desperation to get the better of you. I did, and the results were disastrous. I threw myself at someone, whom I'll call Max, firm in the belief that once he got to know me he'd discover how attractive I really am. This folly lead to nearly a year of subjecting myself to emotional abuse and codependency, which was totally avoidable if I'd followed one simple rule, which I'll get to in a minute.

Looking back, I have no idea what attracted me to Max. I fixated on him, even after I found out he was a drug addict in the midst of a divorce who had actually entered rehab in a last-ditch effort to save his marriage. I pursued him in sometimes embarrassing ways, even though he'd shown no interest in me.

Maybe part of the attraction was that I thought I could "save" him—that my clean lifestyle would set a good example for him as he broke free of drug dependency. I couldn't, and he didn't.

We first met while we were both doing community theater. Max was one of the performers, playing the villain Jigger in the musical *Carousel*. I had no idea how prophetic that would turn out to be. The show's director was teaching me how to design, hang and run lights, which I would go on to do for several years on many productions afterwards.

Prior to and during the run of the show, I was unable to garner much interest from Max. After the show ended, I'd pretty much given up on a relationship ever developing. About two weeks later, he knocked on my door, needing a place to stay for "a night or two." I let him in, flattered that he'd thought of me as someone to come to in a time of need. It turned out that he was looking for someone to take advantage of, and in my loneliness and insecurity I fit the bill perfectly. That night or two turned into nearly a year.

To his credit, Max never pretended to love me, but for those many months I was immobilized by the desire to believe he really could change and by my own fear of being alone again. Even after he moved out at my request, I maintained an irrational level of emotional attachment, and was unable to completely let go. It was only the imminent threat of physical violence that finally convinced me to break free.

What is the simple rule that I did not follow before casting myself in this unhealthy, emotionally destructive relationship? *We did not become friends first.*

Truly, I'm not sure we ever became friends at all. I certainly never considered him my "boyfriend." Rather, even then, I referred to him as my "roommate." In today's parlance, he might be considered a "roommate with benefits," though most definitely he was the one who benefited the most.

I was not a victim, however. I made choices that started this, and I made choices that perpetuated it. Not healthy choices, but mine nonetheless. Yet because I accepted responsibility for my situation, I was eventually also able to make the choices that ultimately ended it, and those choices set my life on a more constructive track.

The idea that you actually have a choice in who gets to be a part of your life is important, and it's an idea that a lot of us don't grasp right away. Sometimes we feel that because our circumstances changed due to things that were not our choice, that our other choices are somehow taken away. Whomever gets to share your life should consider it a privilege, just as you should feel privileged to share theirs. Relationships should be born out of mutual interest and respect.

Back in high school, I'd be walking down the hall and occasionally I'd encounter a group of guys who would eye me as I passed. One would elbow his buddy, point at me, and say something rude like, "There goes your girlfriend!" Even though I knew it was intended as an insult to me for not being "girlfriend material" and to his buddy for allegedly not being able to "do better," one of the thoughts that would cross my mind as I walked away was along the lines of, "Who says I'd want that guy as a boyfriend anyway? Maybe he's not my type." Even through the hurt, I recognized that what *I* wanted in a relationship mattered, too. Even if I did lose sight of that now and again.

I was still doing light design for community theater when I met Ian Shaw. Fresh out of my experience of trying to sustain an unhealthy one-sided relationship with Max, I wasn't particularly looking for a romantic relationship when I met Ian. I was merely continuing to do something I enjoyed. Ian was the primary light tech at a different theater. In the community theater world, there are limited resources, so often people bounce between companies.

The first time we met, Ian had come to "my" theater, where I was lighting a production of *Music Man*. The director knew Ian's work and valued his opinion, so she invited him to come have a look at what I was doing to make sure my design was good. Ian and I were introduced and exchanged pleasantries. My work passed muster, and for me at least, the initial meeting passed from memory. At the time, I was still in the final throes of the Max story, though it was either in or nearing its denouement.

Later that year, a different director invited me to light the musical *Nunsense* at the theater where Ian held the technical board position and did the bulk of his lighting work. This theater was technically much more complex than what I was used to, so I needed Ian's help to create and execute my design.

When you work in technical theater, you need full access to the stage so you can drop bars via the fly system in order to hang lights on them, and move ladders around so you can focus the lights you've been hanging. Out of necessity, you spend a lot of time in the space when there are no rehearsals going on. Many times it was just Ian and me working on weekends and late into the night on and over the stage. As a result, we had a lot of private time to get to know each other.

Our relationship came on gradually. There were no fireworks or flashes of passion. We figured out that we liked each other and had some common interests, so we decided to spend more time together outside of theater. By that time, I was completely over Max. If there had been any overlap, I would not have been ready.

Though we had many lunches and dinners included in our work schedule, our first actual date didn't happen until I invited him to attend the Western Washington State Fair with me, which was in September 1992.

Three years later, we were married.

Ian expressed recently that he wished he'd met me sooner. I think we met just at the right time, as I had some hard but valuable lessons to learn. Maybe meeting Ian would have saved me from an emotionally abusive relationship, but I know that I am a wiser person for having lived through that experience. Not that I recommend it, just as I don't recommend having affairs with men with whom you can't possibly have a lasting relationship. The experiences taught me many things that I can relay so you have a better chance of avoiding them. At the same time, your own experiences will mature you in the ways you'll need to discover yourself.

My face was never an issue for Ian. He valued my other assets, such as creativity, intelligence, work ethic, fiscal responsibility and sense of humor.

Admittedly, it helped that I had (and still have) a shapely figure.

You, too, have attributes that are attractive for both forming friendships as well as romantic relationships. Your interests, areas of expertise, hobbies and experiences are all realms in which you can find common ground with others. I met the love of my life doing community theater, a pastime in which I no longer participate. However, I've made many friends via my current passions: Icelandic horses, being an author, professional speaking, and being a fan and supporter of a handful of independent bands.

If you are doing things you enjoy, and spending time around people who make you happy, you will radiate that joy. You will feel better about yourself, which boosts your self-esteem and your confidence.

Your sense of worth and your happiness should not be based on what anyone else thinks of you. If you are constantly trying to please someone else hoping that they will like you better, then you are compromising your own identity. The best person you can be is yourself. If you like yourself, then it follows that others will like you. You don't have to like your appearance to love who you are on the inside, but it helps if you are at least at peace with it.

If you do meet someone that interests you, be sure to take the time to become friends first. I believe is fundamental to any successful relationship. The romance part may just sneak up on you when you least expect it!

CHAPTER 5: "I CANNOT POSSIBLY LIVE A FULL, HAPPY LIFE."

TAKING CONTROL AND MOVING YOUR WHOLE LIFE FORWARD.

When I learn that someone with a facial difference resists venturing out into the world because they are afraid of the glances, the stares and potential rude comments, my heart hurts for them. They compromise their own happiness because they are so worried about *what others think*.

Moving forward after a dramatic change in your physical appearance is daunting. Reclusion equals security. Inertia equals comfort. Or so it seems.

You may put off finding a job, pursuing an interesting activity, or exploring a relationship because that forces you out of your quiet, safe cocoon. It might be tempting to reject every opportunity with "oh, I *can't.*" Are you throwing up barriers so you can keep it easy for yourself? Effort can be difficult, and sometimes painful. Change often calls forth uncertainty, and you may be finding it difficult to cope with the changes that you are being forced to make. Therefore, you find yourself unwilling to create more change.

You might also be concerned about being stigmatized, or labeled. The non-profit organization B Stigma-Free describes *stigma* as "...the attitude that someone is unacceptable because they are different." Other members of society believe that stigmatized individuals are, among other things, less capable, less intelligent, and less productive. People who are stigmatized may be starting at a disadvantage when it comes to finding a job or having any sort of social interaction.

Be careful not to *self*-stigmatize. Don't buy into the propaganda and believe yourself to be less capable, even if others around you seem to feel that way about you. People assign less value to what they either do not know or understand. But you know what you are capable of, and who you really are, and your integrity to yourself matters.

In his book *Changing Faces*, James Partridge offers this advice as both caution and encouragement: "In rebuilding self-esteem, one thing to your advantage is the pressure to succeed—whatever that might mean—has been lifted as a result of your disfigurement. Your family and your peers will probably reassess your prospects downwards: their ambitions for you will be lowered. But *you* need not lower your ambitions. They may have to be redirected, but as long as your mind and body are still alive—even if disfigured— you stand a chance."

Focus on what you *can* do rather than what you or others think you *can't*.

If for whatever reason you find yourself in a position of needing to get a job, you may feel that your face will place you at a severe disadvantage. While you might have to give a little extra, this disadvantage is not insurmountable. When I queried a group on social media about how having a facial difference affected their ability to interview for a job, the responses I got from participants with actual facial differences indicated it had little or no perceived impact, as long as they went in prepared to emphasize their qualifications.

When you go in for your interview, after exchanging pleasantries, I recommend dispelling the "elephant in the room" right away. Volunteer a brief explanation about your face, and assure the interviewer that it has no affect on your ability to do the job you have applied for. While you are not legally obligated to do any of this, offering an explanation will satisfy the interviewer's inevitable curiosity and lessen the distraction. They will more easily adjust to your appearance if they are told what to make of it, so switching focus to your qualifications will be much more immediate. If your face isn't a big deal to you, it will become less of a big a deal to those who may be seeing it for the first time.

Be positive and optimistic. Act like you're happy to be there (hopefully you really are), and don't forget to smile! Even if you feel your smile isn't so flattering anymore, a smile still lights up your face, radiating happiness and positivity, and those are universal ice-breakers.

If you fail to get the job, it would be easy to jump to the conclusion that your physical appearance may have been a factor. However, there are lots of reasons that people don't get the job they have applied for. For example, you might not have been the best applicant after all. Maybe someone else who applied knows someone who works there, or was referred by them, which gave them an immediate leg up. Maybe someone else was an internal candidate, and they had an advantage due to a policy of promoting from within. Don't assume it's because of your face, and try not to be discouraged.

It might be worth doing a little self-examination and consider whether or not you *really want* the job you are applying for. If the only reason you want it is because you're desperate for the money, you're likely going to be a less convincing candidate than if you want the job because you are incredibly qualified and you think it would be a romping good time. While money can alleviate stress, it is not the key to happiness. Desperation, or even trying too hard, can be off-putting, so please check yourself, your presentation, and your motives when evaluating the feedback you are receiving.

It is conceivable that some managers or companies may be uncomfortable having you doing work that puts you in direct contact with the customer. They have the unfortunate attitude that doing so might hurt the company's image. As backwards as that attitude might be, it is nonetheless out of your control. In situations like these, it is important to remember that interviews work both ways. You are interviewing the company just as much as company management is interviewing you. If there is any hostility or lack of acceptance due to your altered physical appearance, odds are that is not a place that you would want to work anyway. Discovering this during the interview process is an important win, because it spares you a negative experience. They lose out on your wonderfulness, and you don't begin to invest yourself somewhere your talents and abilities won't be appreciated.

My first job out of college was working at a Dairy Queen fast food restaurant. That particular owner had a reputation for hiring people with disabilities of all sorts, and his managers had no problem assigning me to front counter work. As it turned out, I discovered that I didn't have an aptitude for taking orders, but that realization had nothing to do with my face. We all have different strengths and weaknesses. Had I been hidden away in the kitchen or assigned only to bussing tables, I might not have learned that about myself, so I am grateful I had that opportunity. I chose not to be concerned with what the customers thought about my face when I worked at the front counter. In fact, I often didn't give it much thought and didn't hardly notice if customers reacted. I did the best job I could, and if I got their order wrong, I simply fixed it.

Always do your best, and recognize that not every outcome is within your ability to control.

You cannot control how people react to you, but you *can* control your own behavior and how you respond to circumstances. If you are expecting everyone to stare at you, then staring is what you will see. You might even find yourself oddly disappointed if you discover that people are not staring at you. However, the instances of staring will likely make more of an impact on your memory than the times that no one stares.

I am not constantly thinking about my different face, so it's often not forefront in my mind. Usually, I am just thinking about the errand I am running, remembering all the items on my list, or what menu item I feel like eating at that particular restaurant.

When I walk into a place, I do so with the assumption that I am going to be treated like anyone else. I have no expectation that I should be treated in any special way, nor do I expect to be treated disrespectfully. I interact with people in a normal way, and for the most part, I am treated in a normal way. I either don't notice, or don't dwell on, the looks people might give me as they adjust to my appearance. It can be an abrupt reminder that I am unique when my difference is pointed out to me by a stare, a child's curious inquiry, or even an adult's clumsy remark. But we have to learn to brush these encounters off and move on.

You do maintain some control over your appearance. For example, you control your own presentation of poise and posture. If you stand tall, move with confidence and look people in the eye, that will make a very different impression than if you are slumped over, shuffling, and refuse to make eye contact. One way to avoid getting mugged on a city street is to *not* act like a potential victim. Instead, move like someone who shouldn't be messed with, who is aware and observant of their environment, and in control of their destiny.

You also control how you dress, and how you dress can certainly affect how you feel. Since I work from home and live on a small horse farm, I am often wearing barn clothes: worn jeans, T-shirt and a ragged sweatshirt. I am very comfortable in such clothes. When I go out, however, I upgrade my jeans and sweatshirt to something not quite so tattered. When I speak professionally, I don slacks and blouses. In other words, I dress the part. I am not comfortable in skirts or dresses, so only wear them on very special occasions, but even then it's fun to play "dress-up." My point is this: my face does not affect my clothing choices. I choose to be comfortable. I choose to belong. I choose what I wear when, and how I wish to feel in my own clothes.

Poise and attitude trump garb. If you don't believe me, think of examples of people who can wear *anything* and still look good.

You may be able to wear makeup or other cosmetic products to enhance your appearance, or even to camouflage your scars. I generally choose not to, partially because cosmetics do little to mask paralysis, and partially because smearing stuff on my face is not how I choose to spend my time. Plus I am constantly having to dab my watering eye which sometimes drips down my face, causing streaks if I am wearing blush and foundation. But if you are comfortable with putting on makeup or using other camouflaging products to mask your scars, and this allows you feel better about being around other people, go for it. After all, *you* need to figure out what makes you comfortable. When you are comfortable, that is one step closer to happiness.

Regardless of how you choose to go forth into the world, I implore you to do so. Go to a movie. The library. A sporting event. A concert. If you have reservations about going out alone, take a friend who looks "normal" so you not only have an easier time blending in, but someone to interact with as well. That can do much for your confidence in new surroundings and among strangers, and it can also allow you to focus on having a good time rather than tracking the responses that you may receive from people you do not know.

Happiness is not defined by appearance. If it was, then everyone we consider physically attractive would be happy, and that's definitely not the case. Happiness is gained by recognizing your worth, cultivating positive, healthy relationships, and by having a sense of fulfillment. All of this is most certainly within your grasp, even with a facial difference.

Vanessa Carter in South Africa experienced several significant medical setbacks during her long recovery and facial rebuilding process after her car accident. Instead of beating her down, her experiences only steeled her resolve. In her essay, *Six Days*, in which she tells about six independent days that changed her life, she related the following:

> "I was convinced that I might not wake up the next morning. Three months after my minor facial infection, my lower intestines collapsed. I had an adhesive bowel obstruction caused by internal scarring from the accident. I couldn't eat or drink for two weeks, and had pipes feeding food to my body. I was badly ill and in the most severe pain. I lay in bed thinking about what I had done in my life in pursuit of my dreams. I thought about stupid material stuff like that nice sports car I always wanted, the overseas trip I never took, and the things that most of us call *living*. I was only thirty-four and I was lying helpless in a hospital ward beside eighty year old ladies and my mind kept telling me *I shouldn't be here*. It had been nine years since my accident and all I was finding in my life was hospitals, illness, medication, complication, isolation and reasons why I couldn't do the things I really wanted to do. It took me eight weeks

to recover. During that time, I cultivated the mindset that I would never waste another day of my life."

Vanessa is currently leading a revolution in online patient communication and advocacy. She discovered her mission and is following her passion.

After being severely burned in Iraq, JR Martinez's positive attitude about his changed appearance prompted nurses to ask him to talk to other burn patients who were having a harder time coping with their own physical changes. JR discovered how helpful this connection and mentorship was, not only for those other patients, but for himself as well. He embarked on a journey that led him to become an actor, author, motivational speaker, and even the 2011 season winner of *Dancing with the Stars*. He is an advocate for injured veterans as well as spokesperson for several charitable organizations including Operation Finally Home, the Phoenix Society for Burn Survivors, and Iraq and Afghanistan Veterans of America.

You don't have to lead a revolution like Vanessa, or become a celebrity like JR to continue leading a fulfilling life. Just go out and do things that give you a sense of accomplishment. Activities that make you feel *alive*. Do what you loved before anything changed in your life. Experiment with new interests, too. Take lessons. Volunteer. Surround yourself with people who have similar interests, and whose company you enjoy. People who build you up rather than tear you down.

Be a good listener. There will be many who have advice for you, and only you can decide which of it you want to take. No one else can change you, but they can open your mind to new possibilities. Be discerning of the motives and sincerity of people, and at the same time be open to receiving love and support. It may come from places you never expect.

Sure, life may have thrown you a curve ball. It's your choice if you want to swing for the fences or just stand there and watch it go by.

It's not easy facing the world every day with a face that isn't perfect. But then, life isn't easy for anyone, and your face was probably never perfect anyway.

"One of the basic rules of the universe is that nothing is perfect. Perfection simply doesn't exist...
without imperfection, neither you nor I would exist."
—Stephen Hawking

Happiness is a choice. You choose how you want to go forward with your life. You can stagnate in uncertainty, indecision and fear, or you can march forward to new adventures and new challenges.

CONCLUSION: EMBRACING YOUR IDENTITY

Society seems to want to cast those of us who are different into one of two roles: bitter and unhappy because we've been dealt a difficult hand, or brave and inspirational because of how *well* we've come through our adverse experiences. As you know, life isn't as clear-cut as all that. There's a lot of gray in between.

Confusion, guilt, insecurity, loneliness, frustration, hurt—you are going to continue to experience all of these unpleasant feelings at times. Hopefully you are also able to add positive emotions like pride, acceptance, accomplishment, success, love and friendship to your list, and the warmth and light these experiences give you will stave off the frigid periods of darkness.

People will call you *brave.*

When people call me "brave," I accept it as a compliment, even though it puzzles me. I am pretty sure they are referring to that fact that I go out into the world every day and live a full life with a different face, but for me, the alternative is unthinkable. I would not want to limit my opportunities and experiences by hiding myself away.

Perhaps people assume that we must deal with stares, questions, comments and taunts on a daily basis. Periodically, yes—but fortunately for me at least, this is not a daily experience. Out of necessity, we learn to adjust.

I choose to go out into the world and live my life. How is that *brave,* exactly?

Perhaps I am considered brave because I speak publicly to both kids and adult groups about developing resilience, as well as accepting and embracing differences in both themselves and others. I'm comfortable speaking to groups, and it's important to me to get my message out. So still I ask, how is that brave? Because I take the risk that I will not be accepted? So does everyone else.

One of my *Friending the Mirror* webinar guests, musician Kit Karlson, was struck with Bell's Palsy the day before he was scheduled to go on an intense three-week tour with his band, Stephen Kellogg and the Sixers. With half his face suddenly and inexplicably paralyzed, activities like eating, speaking and smiling were adversely affected. He elected to go on the tour anyway. [Find a link to the interview with Kit and view the complete list of webinar episodes at www.facinguptoit.com/webinar.]

During our interview, I called him "brave." What's the difference? Why is he brave and not me?

It's not about humility. I've been this way all my life. In terms of my face and my personality, I don't know any differently. I know that my appearance doesn't affect my ability to do almost anything I want to do, and I am very grateful for that. I've had speech therapy, and while I am not the tidiest eater, I've adapted. I've also adapted to the stares, questions, and reactions of people around me as I move into new situations. In some respects, I take these things for granted. These are my "norm."

For Kit, however, this was all a new experience thanks to the sudden onset of Bell's. The choice for him to go on tour was easy; for him it was primarily because he didn't want to let his band down. His skill on the keyboard was unaffected, even if he did have to give up playing the tuba for a time. As stressful as the tour was, he was at least sheltered by the support of his band mates, friends and fans.

In retrospect, Kit admitted that doing the tour was the best thing for him. It prevented him from holing up in his house and feeling sorry for himself, worrying about how long the Bell's Palsy might last.

Also, once his situation was known within his circles, he came to realize that quite a few people have had experience with Bell's Palsy, either personally or via someone they know. He was luckier than many. His symptoms only lasted two weeks.

Did he endure stares? Yes. Did he have trouble eating? Absolutely! As a result, he kept to himself during meals. Did he smile on stage? I'm sure he did. And while it wasn't his usual smile, his smile still conveyed the same meaning to anyone looking on.

Bravery is being afraid and doing it anyway. Kit had a lot of unknowns to be afraid of, because this experience was completely new to him. He actually was afraid, and yet he faced that fear and went on tour anyway. Hence, Kit was brave.

You may be afraid at first, and if you face those fears and carry on, then you truly are *brave*. But when it comes to our faces, there shouldn't be any reason to be afraid.

People will call you *inspirational*. This can be difficult to accept, and you might resist this label, too, because you certainly didn't ask for this challenge. If you feel you are not worthy of admiration, or if you feel you are being put up on a pedestal, I can understand the discomfort.

How should you respond when someone says to you *"You're such an inspiration?"* Start by saying *"thank you."* Like being called *brave,* I choose to take being called "an inspiration" as a compliment.

There is nothing wrong with being an inspiration. The definition of *inspiration* is "the action or power of moving the intellect or emotions; a person, place, experience, etc. that makes someone want to do or create something." Being an inspiration means being the force or influence that inspires someone to do something or to feel a certain way. In most uses, the person bestowing this designation means it in a very positive way.

I enjoy being that force. I am grateful that my own story and experiences have empowered me to influence people, and to encourage them to embrace their differences and make choices that help them live happier lives. That's why I put myself out there, writing books and speaking professionally. However, being an inspiration means you wouldn't want others to view what you have as unobtainable. Instead, you want the people you inspire to feel that they can achieve what you have, or a version of it authentic to themselves. You want to instigate the mindset *"If she can do it, so can I!"*

And it's OK if you need a little help. I know I did. It took time to grow into this identity, and that was an authentic part of my journey. In some ways, needing and receiving help is what inspired me to write and speak to others in the way I reach out today.

If you can set an example through your positive choices, success, survival, happiness, confidence or whatever, how is that a bad thing? If you can inspire someone to aspire to a happier, more active, more productive life, isn't that what any of us could hope for?

Don't let your altered face define you, but embrace it as part of your identity. It will teach you a lot about yourself, and about human nature, if you let it. It won't all be pleasant, but it will all be valuable. There will be setbacks and disappointments. There always are in any aspect of life.

You don't have to be happy, confident and upbeat all the time. I'd worry about you if you were. I certainly don't always feel as confident as people perceive me to be. You are allowed to be human. However, like the balance in a bank account, keep the positive ahead of the negative. Look for ways to attain positive when you are feeling negative. It is your responsibility to replenish your account when you run empty.

You are not alone. If you are looking for a support community, contact me and I'll put you in touch.

Recognize that love is possible. Anyone who cannot see past your appearance is not worthy of you.

Most importantly, get out into the world and never let anyone forget that there is a person behind the face. You may have new challenges and the learning curve to manage them may be sharp, but you are still fundamentally the same person you always were. You can still do things you enjoy, and you can even try new things. Don't let anyone stop you, and especially don't get in your own way.

Choose happiness. Light up the world with your asymmetrical smile.

REFERENCES

Publications:

Changing Faces, by James Partridge

The Church of 80% Sincerity, David Roche

"Six Days," an essay by Vanessa Carter. (Published as "Everything Happens for a Reason" in *Chocolate and Diamonds for the Woman's Soul* by Hot Pink Publishing, 2015)

An Inside Look at Being Outside of Ordinary, by Charlene Pell, founder of Facing Forward, Inc.

Survival of the Prettiest, the Science of Beauty by Nancy Etcoff- quoted by Charlene Pell in her article *An Inside Look at Being Outside of Ordinary*

Daring Greatly by Brené Brown

Internet:

Facial Discrimination, by Neil Steinberg. First published with Mosaic http://mosaicscience.com/ republished here under a Creative Commons license. View article in its entirety at http://mosaicscience.com/story/faces

Changing Faces http://changingfaces.org.uk/ and their self help guides https://www.changing-faces.org.uk/Adults/Self-help-guides

5 Ways to Escape Your Victim Mentality - Emily Roberts, MA LPC Posted November 1, 2012 on http://www.healthyplace.com/blogs/buildingselfesteem/2012/11/5-ways-to-escape-your-victim-mentality/

Friending the Mirror webinar series http://www.facinguptoit.com/webinar/

BStigmaFree http://bstigmafree.org/

The Adults with Facial Differences Networking Community on Facebook

RESOURCES

Publications:

Changing Faces, by James Partridge. http://changing-faces.org.uk/

The Church of 80% Sincerity, by David Roche. http://www.davidroche.com/

Full of Heart: My Story of Survival, Strength and Spirit by JR Martinez. http://jrmartinez.com/

Life with Scars by Brady Armstrong. www.rarecases.com

Internet

Changing Faces' self help guides https://www.changingfaces.org.uk/Adults/Self-help-guides

Facing Forward, Inc. http://www.facingforwardinc.org/

AboutFace http://www.aboutface.ca/

Phoenix Society for Burn Survivors http://www.phoenix-society.org/

Moebius Syndrome Foundation http://moebiussyndrome.org/

Friending the Mirror webinar series http://www.facinguptoit.com/webinar/

BStigmaFree http://bstigmafree.org/

The Adults with Facial Differences Networking Community on Facebook

The Physical Differences Support, Discussion and Advocacy Group on Facebook

Facial Discrimination, by Neil Steinberg. http://mosaicscience.com/story/faces

ACKNOWLEDGMENTS

Ian Shaw, my extraordinary husband, who indulges me in most of my projects.

Charlene Pell, founder of Facing Forward, Inc., for generously sharing her research on "Why People Stare."

James Partridge, for allowing me to use pieces of his amazing book *Changing Faces*, which inspired the foundation of his non-profit organization of the same name in the United Kingdom.

All my amazing guests on my *Friending the Mirror* webinar series who so openly share their knowledge, stories and experiences live on the internet in the interest of helping and inspiring others. Visit www.facinguptoit.com/webinar for a complete list.

Kate Makled, my coach and editor, and all my friends and fellow authors who have supported the creation of this publication.

Ellen Violette, for helping me bring *Facial Shift* to print.

ABOUT THE AUTHOR

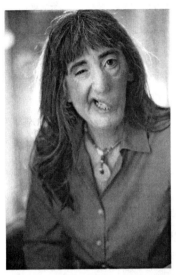

Professional motivational speaker Dawn Shaw understands adversity and embodies resilience, which she believes is the key to bully-resistance. She was born with a rare tumor, the removal of which left her face half paralyzed, so she grew up looking "different." Despite the insecurities and unfair treatment this sometimes brings, she learned to accept and even embrace her difference and lives a happy and productive life.

Her inspiring memoir *Facing Up to It*, published in early 2013, shares her stories and experiences during her challenging journey to confidence and self-acceptance. Her second book, a Kindle exclusive titled *Friending the Mirror; Changing How You See Your Reflection*, is a guide to finding beauty through happiness. She currently hosts an online video series, also titled *Friending the Mirror,* in which guests educate and share their personal stories about appearance-related issues and insecurities, disabilities, and physical differences. She has taken her inspiring message to television by appearing on an episode of the Discovery Channel's *Body Bizarre,* which will air in 2016.

When not writing or speaking to youth or adult groups about such topics as developing resilience, accepting and embracing differences and the value of diversity, Dawn indulges in her affinity for live music, attending concerts primarily by independent rock bands with Ian, her husband of over 20 years. She also runs a small Icelandic horse farm in western Washington, which is home to several well-loved cats and dogs and an ever-changing number of Icelandic horses. For more information on Dawn and how she influences her world, visit www.facinguptoit.com.

THANK YOU OFFER FOR READERS

SPECIAL OFFER!

Visit www.facinguptoit.com to download an audio version of her Kindle eBook *Friending the Mirror*, a how-to guide on developing resilience by finding beauty through happiness.

Dawn Shaw is a Professional Motivational Speaker.

Dawn is an expert on resilience, which she believes is the key to becoming bully-resistant. Youth and adult audiences alike are drawn in by her openness in sharing her personal stories about living with a facial difference. Her direct, engaging and entertaining style compels the audience toward accepting and embracing differences in themselves and others as well as learning how they, too, can become more resilient.

What people are saying about Dawn's presentations:

> "Dawn helps students develop understanding
> for and appreciation of people with differences
> instead of making fun of them."
> —Andrew Smallman | Director, Puget Sound
> Community School, Seattle, WA

> "Dawn's talk far exceeded expectations. She
> blew the veil off a sensitive topic and helped
> give much better perspective on people
> who may generally appear to be physically
> different. Several members of our Club have
> approached me since her talk to say how much
> they appreciated her message."
> —Victor Ulsh, Program Chairman, East
> Bremerton Rotary

Visit http://www.facinguptoit.com/speaking/ for information, testimonials and booking.

For a short video demonstration of Dawn's power of engagement, view:

on YouTube https://www.youtube.com/watch?v=-FSygsl9jwQ

on Wistia https://facinguptoit.wistia.com/medias/1615i0jif5

on Vimeo https://vimeo.com/149723497

Want to read more? Look for Dawn's memoir, *Facing Up to It,* available in print and eBook formats, and her Kindle eBook, *Friending the Mirror* at http://www.facinguptoit.com/books/

Find Dawn on Twitter @facinguptoit https://twitter.com/facinguptoit

and Facebook www.facebook.com/facinguptoit

CPSIA information can be obtained
at www.ICGtesting.com
Printed in the USA
FSOW02n1617060416
18827FS